THE Spa BIBLE

The Gospel On Starting YOUR OWN Spa Business

Bestselling Author
CANDACE HOLYFIELD

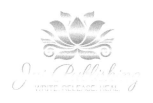

Copyright © 2019 by Candace Holyfield

All rights reserved. No part of this publication may be reproduced, distributed, or transmitted in any form or by any means, including photocopying, recording, or other electronic or mechanical methods, without the prior written permission of the publisher, except in the case of brief quotations embodied in critical reviews and certain other noncommercial uses permitted by copyright law. For permission requests, write to the publisher, addressed "Attention: Permissions Coordinator," at the address below.

Jai Publishing, Inc.
Website: www.jaipublishing.com
Email: info@jaipublishing.com

Printed in the United States of America

ISBN-13: 9781077120181

Dedication

For my kids:
Mahogany, Jorden, & Brooklyn

I love you all so much! Each of you have given me the strength to build a legacy for our family!

This one is for ALL of you!

Contents

In The Beginning v

Genesis 3

Disciples 21

Numbers 28

Chronicles 36

Job 50

Acts 57

Revelation 65

Spa Law 71

Acknowledgments 81

INTRODUCTION

In The Beginning...

Let There Be Groupon

I was seven months pregnant, headed to work at Massage Envy, the spa where I worked at that time. My car ran hot, and I decided to quit my job that day.

Months prior to my pregnancy, I submitted a request for my deal to be featured on Groupon and was told they could not help me at that time.

A few weeks after I quit my job, Groupon decided they wanted to do business with me. My deal was LIVE on their platform within a few days after signing my contract.

It was selling like hot cakes!

I made over $6,000 in 3 days. It was my first time in life making that amount of money in such a short period of time.

I went into labor while my deal was featured all over Groupon. I thought I could return to work in two weeks, but my c-section quickly informed me that my body was not ready.

Seeing that my body was recouping from giving birth to my child, my mom along with a good friend became my team.

And there you have it, just like that... I went from making $15 at Massage Envy to running my OWN spa, with a team, within 30 days!

With my newfound business in tow, a new baby, and a healing body, I quickly learned how to master running a business. Needless to say, my business expanded and so did my team.

My years in running my spa business taught me a great deal. I have made a lot of money, and at times, I lost a lot too.

I have worked with tons of celebrities, sold thousands of ebooks and courses all over the world, graced the pages of American Spa Magazine and created the dopest spa professionals community (Spa Boss Tribe), all while building two six-figure brands that I love: Candy Spa Parties and 6 Figure Spa Chick!

In this book, I am sharing how I have sustained the last six years as 100% entrepreneur.

Just so that you know, the material I share in this book has helped me:

- ◆ Support a rebooking rate of 9 out of 10;

- ◆ Make over $100k in sales from Groupon;

- ◆ Leverage social media to build my brand, with Instagram as my #1 marketing tool;

- ◆ Generate my first 100k in sales WITHOUT Groupon;

- ◆ Create passive income while continuing to grow my spa revenue;

... And so much more!

I invite you on this journey—whether you are brand new to the spa business, or you have a spa business that you would like to improve.

I didn't always get it right, but I did get me HERE. And that's a reason to celebrate!

Love,

Candace

Six Figure Spa Chick

THE Spa BIBLE

The Gospel On Starting YOUR OWN Spa Business

Bestselling Author
CANDACE HOLYFIELD

CHAPTER I

Genesis

Let There Be Spa

⇒ ⇒ ⇒ Critical Steps to Starting YOUR Spa Business

You MUST have a plan even before you start your spa business. That is the biggest mistake that most spa business owners make—they plan as they go and therefore, they are moving by the seat of their pants instead of being prepared for things as they occur.

From my experience, here are some critical steps to starting your own spa. Make sure you take the time to sort through these steps as they will definitely set you up to have success within your own spa.

Determine the services you are going to offer.

This is important so that you can identify the competition in your area and be able to figure out your final profit.

Each service has an amount that it costs to service the client. The rest is your profit. You must know in advance which services are going to pay the bills and which services are extra.

Remember that in order to be considered a spa, you must offer at least two of the three following services:

- massage
- skin care OR
- body treatments

Consider what equipment you need in advance.

Some services require more equipment and more utilities—for instance water and special plumbing for hydrotherapy, so you may want to introduce more inexpensive services first and then ramp up to more expensive services.

As your business generates more cash, you can then invest in the special, or more expensive equipment as well as pay the extra utilities. Scaling is key!

Failing to scale services may cost you your business because you will not be able to remain profitable if you are putting all of your money in expensive equipment first.

The look and feel of the spa will decide on what type of customers you want to attract.

Many people ONLY think luxury spa when they are contemplating opening a spa; however, nowadays, people are looking for the UBER of different services. Some people may be happy with less fluff if they get to attend the spa more often because the pricing is budget friendly.

You can also consider things like a male only spa, an organic ingredients spa, or any other type of trending new age spa that meets current consumer demands.

Now this level of services automatically puts you in a totally different market than your competitors!

Consider your location carefully.

This also has a lot to do with what services you offer and the look and feel of the spa. If you are in a primarily student area, you may scale BACK on looks in order to offer something that is budget conscious.

If you are in a medical center area, then price may not be as important as the ability to have access to services that get them in and out quickly. (Remember that medical professionals have a small window of time between their work shifts.)

Or, in the case of nurses and doctors that stay on their feet all day, do you offer foot massages? Again, consider the geographic location and the businesses that operate in that vicinity.

The more you know about the area you are putting your spa in, the more successful you will be.

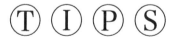

Visit your new spa home on the weekends and at night so you can get a feel for the area during the off hours.

> Identify potential issues, like parking and safety, that may drive people away. It is great to align your spa with stores like Wal-Mart and Target that also gives you the 'walk-by' exposure.

> Steer clear of industrial areas and office building areas where the business tends to die off after 5:00 p.m.

Consider your operating hours.

Just like the things we've already covered, you can't decide your operating hours based on when YOU want to work. You must decide your operating hours based on when YOUR clients need you to be available.

Here again is an opportunity to get more business by being different.

For example, if you serve the medical community, consider being open super early and occasionally super late.

Maybe you open 7 days a week or only 6. But allow all of this to be dictated by who you serve, or you may find yourself with no one to serve.

Decide how much space you will need.

EVEN if you will not START with all of your initial offerings, it is easier to add-on IF you have the space. Once you are out of space, you are out of options.

Visit other spas to see how to maximize the space in your spa. Remember, the more you are able to do within your space, without increasing your monthly rent, the more profit you will receive.

Keep in mind things like:

- Waiting Areas
- Post Treatment Areas
- Retail Offerings
- Salon Services
- Treatment Rooms
- Consultation Rooms
- Office Space
- Employee Break-rooms and Lockers
- Client Breakrooms and Lockers
- Changing Rooms

- Storage

- Restrooms

While you may be able to have some of these areas serve double duty, such as the bathroom and changing area, you also want to make sure you don't lose whatever ambiance you are working to create.

If possible, don't hesitate to consult an architect, a design company or a professional organizer who may be able to shed light on more efficient ways to get more done with less space.

Decide what products you will offer.

Whether you create your own products, offer a well-established brand, or even decide to white label your products, you have to remember that add-on products are a critical part of the profits for your salon business.

Getting your clients into the habit of buying products from you from day one, means you need to start to carry some of their favorite brands as soon as you open the doors.

Again, don't be afraid to visit other spas to see what offerings they have, how they are displayed, how they are priced, and how they are marketed to customers.

The more homework you do, the more you will be equipped to generate profits from products when your salon opens.

Create the right ambience from start to finish.

This means thinking about every aspect of your business even before you open the doors.

⇨ Will your clients have enough locker space? Think about rainy areas where clients will often have umbrellas or cold areas where they may come in with winter coats.

⇨ Are your treatment rooms soundproof? If your clients in the waiting area can HEAR other clients, they won't be comfortable with their own treatments.

Offer products that not only smell great, but have a packaging that matches the décor and ambiance of your spa. Use the products yourself so that you can refer to them when clients ask "What's that smell?"

Invest in quality equipment that is the right height, width and has suitable padding and comfort levels for your clients. Consider plus-sized customers and know that no one wants to lay down on a thinly padded treatment table.

It's okay to start small and build quality versus starting cheap and having to start over and/or risk losing business.

Adjustable lighting and music in each room is important.

You want to be able to adjust lights and music to the client's taste, not just what is playing at the time.

Again, make sure your music and lighting selections are in line with the mood that you want to convey.

Don't overlook adjustable temperatures if possible. People are naturally cold natured or warm natured and one temperature may not fit all depending on what treatment they are receiving.

CHAPTER II

Disciples

Let There Be Team

⇛ ⇛ ⇛ Building a Team for Your Business

Even Jesus had a team! So no matter what type of salon you are opening, there is no way you can operate without a team.

I was blessed to leverage my friends and family in my early days, but that is not always possible.

I also made some mistakes by not being prepared with what to offer my spa employees, and in some cases, I overpaid my employees. I didn't consider the bills before I shared profits with them.

Here are some things you can do to make sure you don't make the same mistakes that I did while building your "disciples" also known as your team:

1. What type of training will you provide? While your spa associates probably have experience in the spa you may want to make sure each of them

receives the following bare minimum treatment from you:

- What your vision and expectations are for YOUR spa

- The repercussions of NOT following YOUR spa rules

- Cross-training on different spa positions, if possible

- Yearly training on changed laws, health ordinances, and industry standards

- Customer service training for YOUR spa

- Emergency procedures for YOUR spa

- Equipment and process Training

- Product and upsells training

- Team building and communication

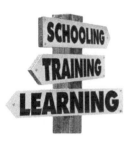

2. Who will you hire? Of course you have to hire spa technicians and people to provide the services you offer, however you must also consider:

- Who will answer the phones and set bookings?

- Who will keep the spa cleaned?

- Who will provide maintenance for the spa?

- Who will complete inventory and replenish products?

- Who will keep the books and report profits?

- Who will complete employee work schedules?

- Who is responsible for marketing spa specials?

- Who is responsible for Web maintenance?

Disciples ... 26

- Who is responsible for social media marketing?

- Who is responsible for the guest experience and handling complaints?

- Who is responsible for employee relationships?

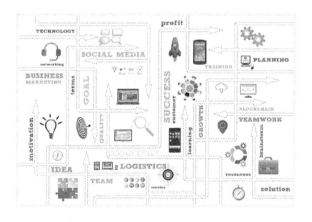

You may be tempted to put YOURSELF next to all of these tasks. It's best you don't.

Consider the things that are most important to the profitability of your business and focus on those.

The more profits you bring in, the more you can afford to spend on employing experts to do the rest.

Make the MAIN thing the MAIN thing and don't hesitate to ask employees to do double duty, especially as you are getting started.

Your spa's success has much to do with the consistency of your team. The spa business is known for a high turnover rate, so the more you engage, train and communicate with your team, the more you can employ and retain quality employees.

CHAPTER III

Numbers

Let There Be Profit

⇒ ⇒ ⇒ **Start-up Money**

It is no doubt that you will need MONEY to start your new business. Here are some popular sources of funding:

☞ YOURSELF ☜

Don't hesitate to work a part-time job or find another way to generate extra revenue while you are working to build the finances for your spa.

Remember the more money you have, the more options you have.

☞ YOUR FAMILY ☜

While it may not always be ideal to borrow money from your family, you may have the opportunity to offer them limited partnership in your business until you pay them back their initial investor money.

Approach them like you would a bank, with your plan in hand and an opportunity for them to earn interest when you pay them back.

After all, they don't OWE you anything.

☞ THE SMALL BUSINESS ADMINISTRATION (SBA) ☜

The SBA has several options for you to provide revenue for your business.

☞ LENDERS ☜

There are lenders that you can google that offer financing specifically for spas and salons, so make sure you take a look for those loans specifically.

☞ MY BOOK: BUSINESS CREDIT 101 ☜

I also have a book on the way to increase your credit and secure business funding for those of you who may not have the best credit.

You can get more information at https://payhip.com/candaceholyfield

Keeping Up With Your Business Money

One of the BIGGEST mistakes spa owners make is that the money is coming in so quickly, they fail to track it. By tracking it, you can TRULY see where your money is coming and going.

At a bare minimum, you should be tracking:

- ☑ Revenue made

- ☑ Product Upsells/Added Revenue

- ☑ Payroll

- ☑ Monthly Recurring Expenses (Lease, Lights, Business Phone, Etc.)

- ☑ Emergency Purchases

As soon as you can hire a business tax professional so that you can focus on building the business. A business tax professional can also help you understand which of your purchases are tax deductible for example marketing, business education (coaches and books and more.

Investing in Your Business

Before you go spending your spa profits to upgrade your lifestyle, or take that long-awaited vacation, consider spending your money by investing back into your spa.

- Add some new services to your spa;

- Buy additional spa equipment that you may not have added when you started;

- Upgrade the ambiance in your spa;

- Add additional products to offer your clients more product diversity and further enhance your bottom line upsells;

- Create sales bonus opportunities for your spa associates to encourage upsells and repeat bookings; or

- Upgrade your web or phone equipment to increase level of automation, allowing you more time to work in your spa.

CHAPTER IV

Chronicles

Let there be Clients

⇛ ⇛ ⇛ Getting Exposure for Your Business

After all of the work you have done to open your business, unfortunately your job is not done.

Many business owners think like field of dreams, if you build it, they will come. Even the most beautiful spa is nothing if no one knows about it. In fact, getting exposure starts long before your spa even opens!

Be creative in reaching out to friends, local media and others to spread the word about your new spa. Build excitement about the spa in spa interests groups and through community newspaper— even before the spa opens.

Have a community-based grand opening event, and make it meaningful and fun for the community to come and SEE you.

These are just the basics of getting exposure before you open, however, once you open your spa, consider yearly special interests events to keep the exposure going.

Possibly free treatments for cancer survivors during Breast Cancer Awareness month or for domestic violence victims during Domestic Violence Awareness months.

The sky is the limit on these events, just make sure they are highly attended and publicized both online and off.

Marketing

Marketing and customer care are arguably the MOST important pieces for the survival of your business.

Here are the most critical pieces for your marketing.

....
For the complete list of marketing do's and don'ts for the spa business, consider investing in my SPAPRENEURS A-Z Guide to Marketing available on Amazon.
....

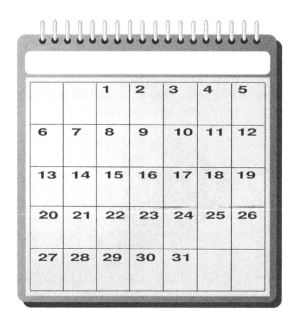

⇒ A Marketing Calendar

Planning activities that bring customers into the door should be done at least one month in advance, if not one year.

Things like National Spa Day and other National Wellness days should be recognized in your spa, as well as other days that are significant according to your spa niche.

⇛ Community Coupon Programs

Services like Groupon go a long ways towards getting you that first round of clients through the door. Even though you may not make much money from the initial visit, your ability to get them to come back will build your profits over time.

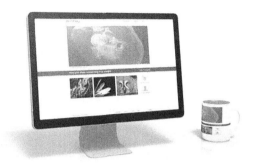

⇛Online

Make sure your website is always updated and that you pay attention to community rating sites such as yelp. Make sure your basic information is updated on Google. Be EASY to find online. Keep your specials updated and make sure clients have the ability to book from your website.

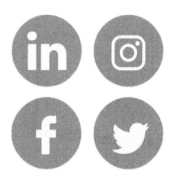

⇛Social Media

The invention of social media has made it easier for businesses to get noticed without huge advertising budgets, but you will have to be creative.

Consider awarding customers who post about their spa visits, because LIKE attracts LIKE. Make sure that you have someone posting daily updates on all of your primary social media platforms such as Facebook, Instagram and Pinterest, and at least a couple times a week on platforms like Linked In.

When you don't post updates, it looks as if your business is abandoned—and it actually is abandoned... ONLINE.

-⚛-

Client Retention

It's cheaper to keep your customers coming back versus finding new ones. Here are some ways you can retain the customers you do have.

Chapter IV

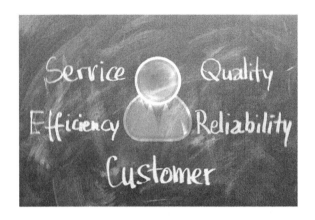

Customer Loyalty Cards

☆☆☆☆

Enticing them with a free or reduced price service upon completion upon a required number of visits or services is a great way to keep them coming back.

Ask for Feedback

Having anonymous surveys or even asking customers for their direct feedback and then USING what they say is a great way to make sure customers KNOW that their feedback is important

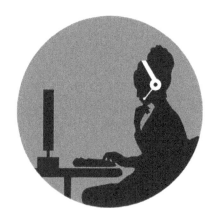

Customer Service

☆ ☆ ☆ ☆

Yes, I know it seems basic, but it's not just about your service. From the time the customer comes into the door, until the time they leave, EVERYONE needs to defer to the customer.

In a day and age where great customers service is so hard to find, you will stand out head and tails above the rest if everyone is extremely helpful and nice. If they can pull it off at a chicken sandwich restaurant, surely you can do it consistently in your spa.

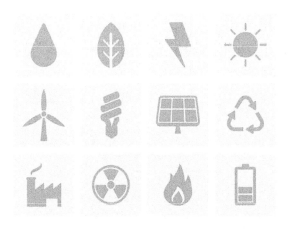

Cleanliness

I know this seems to be another basic element, but again this is not about you... it's about enforcing your standard of excellence even when you are not around.

It doesn't take too many times to get caught slipping on health and hygiene for your spa to build a bad reputation. The easiest way to get rid of a bad reputation is to NEVER develop one in the first place.

CHAPTER V

Job

There Will Be Troubles

⇒ ⇒ ⇒ Managing Tough Times in your Spa Business

There are several things you can do in the spa business to be able to survive the tough times. In EVERY business, times get tough and it can't be avoided but you CAN survive!

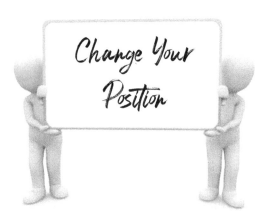

Often times people look at the spa as a luxury and when tough times happen, people often forego luxury in order to make ends meet.

BUT if you frame your spa treatment as WELLNESS and necessary to reduce stress or live a healthier lifestyle, then people can "justify" to themselves the need to go to the spa.

Remember people always have money for what's important to them.

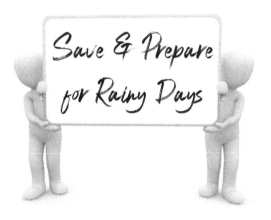

The spa business, depending on your area, can also have seasonal downturns that can be expected based on local trends. You should expect these and make sure employees are aware of them as well.

By planning properly, you and your employees will definitely be prepared both financially and mentally for economic ebbs and flows.

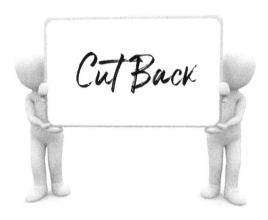

Cut back on higher end treatments – if the demand for higher end treatments slows down, then cut them back and focus on marketing the services that are most in demand.

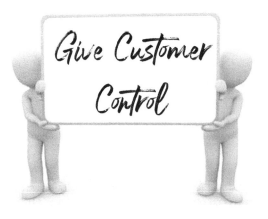

Consider things like loyalty programs and memberships where customers only pay one time a month for a set number of services.

Just like gym memberships, most customers will never redeem all of their services.

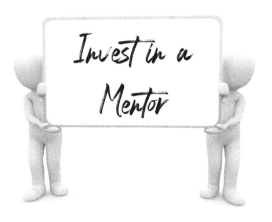

Staying on top of your Spa Study, consider investing in a mentor who has been there (bad times) before. And if you are smart, you will do it BEFORE the bad times come!

It is up to you to stay educated on Spa Trends and to even investigate and copy what other spas may be doing to stay afloat during tough economic times.

There is nothing like other peoples' knowledge. If there is a system that works, use it, but make sure it fits in with YOUR spa goals and mission.

CHAPTER VI

Acts

Let Thy Be Diligent in Leadership

Your spa will be as successful as your leadership. Let's talk characteristics of a successful leader.

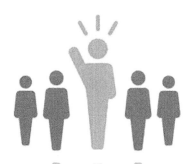

Make Team Building a Priority

The stronger the TEAM, the stronger the business.

Host regular team building exercises for the team, particularly during down time seasons.

Team building teaches trust within the team, and it shows when customers come through the door.

Chapter VI

A team that gets along with each other produces an environment that promotes wellness and good energy. And this is the type of environment and service that attracts more customers.

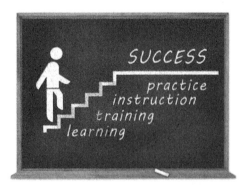

Train, Train, Train

First, find employees that will eventually WANT to start their own spa businesses because they will be the most coachable.

Then make sure that they are getting the necessary training, and even training each other during down time.

Yes, they may eventually leave, but while they are there, you have a fully invested employee instead of someone who's only in it for the 'now' and the money.

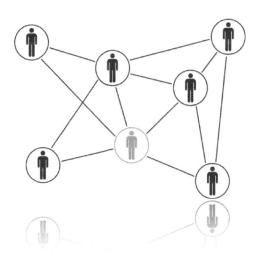

Delegate Your Weakness

The BIGGEST waste of time is trying to do something you are not good at to save a few coins.

Devote YOUR time to VIP sessions and high end tasks that you are good at doing. This will position you to EARN the money to invest in the things you need to delegate.

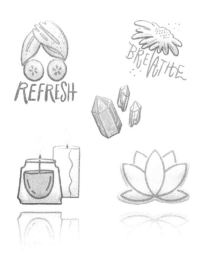

Be CUSTOMER Focused

I can't say enough that the greatest spa in the world makes clients FEEL the greatest.

It's amazing how well having bottled waters, a glass of wine, or fruit infused water can go over in making the customer experience.

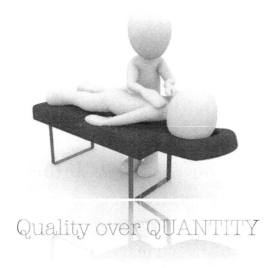

Quality over QUANTITY

You would rather have ONE amazing sold out location than

two lackluster half empty locations. Before you expand make sure you can keep the service elevated at each location.

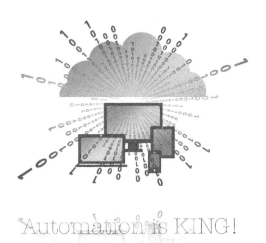

Automation is KING!

Look for ways to automate processes to free you up to spend more time with your customers, your team and marketing.

Look for software and mobile apps dedicated specifically to spas so that you get the best bang for your buck.

CHAPTER VII

Revelation

Let There Be Processes

⇛ ⇛ ⇛ Creating Consistency Through Processes

Nobody really likes a lot of rules, however having them in place means that no one ever has to guess about where you stand on a particular subject.

Having a process in place means that you empower your employees to take care of you, the salon AND your customers in your absence. In the case of emergencies you are better off having your team prepared versus guessing what to do.

Here are some things that you MUST not only create a process for, but also periodically remind your team about.

1. **Day-to-Day Processes**

    a. Opening Process

    b. Closing Process

c. Cleaning Process

d. Cell Phone Policy

e. Social Media Policy

f. Training Policy

g. Customer Refund Policy

2. **Weather Emergency Procedures:** Yeah you may not be in Kansas, but a weather emergency could pop up any day. Your team needs to know how to direct clients in case of:

a. Floods

b. Tornadoes

c. Earthquakes

d. Snowstorms/Blizzards

3. **Robbery Procedures:** Yeah, we hope you NEVER have to use this one, but you never know so it's best to have the policy in place.

   a. How and when to contact the police/authorities

   b. How and when to contact you

   c. How to handle employees

   d. How to handle clients

e. How to secure the salon

4. **Handling Upset/Irate Customers**

5. **How To Contact YOU at all Times in Case of Emergency**

6. **Who Is Next in Charge in YOUR Absence**

Your SOP, or standard operating procedure, manual should include EVERYTHING you can think of and be a liquid document that you add to whenever you come up with a potential situation.

Makes sure your employees are made aware weekly as to updates and how to handle themselves in specific situations. You can thank me later!

CHAPTER VIII

Spa Law

Let There Be SPA

⇛ ⇛ ⇛ 9 Commandments of the Spa Business

LAW #1: Lacking Identity/Branding

If YOU don't know who you are, then you will NOT attract the right clients. Everything, from your logo to the products you sell, TELL people what your brand stands for. Make sure it's consistent.

⇓

LAW #2: Failing to Complete Market Research

Later is too late when it comes to Market Research. Don't wait until you have signed a 12-month lease to figure out that you are in a dead foot traffic area, or that the building next door cooks Thai food that permeates your building with a BAD odor. That's far too late.

⇓

LAW #3: Not Having an Online Presence and Online Booking Ability

Welcome to the 21st century—an age of cell phones and web sites. If you don't make it easy for customers to book with you, they will book with someone else. End of Story.

⇓

LAW #4: Not Making Sales a Priority

Anything that gets in the way of your sales, from booking clients to close, to not making a connection or next appointment while they are already IN the salon, is a detriment.

YOU are in the spa business. If you don't sell products and services consistently and make sure your team is doing the same, you won't last too long. There is simply too much competition.

⇓

LAW #5: Not Focusing on Wellness

Luxury is well and good, but wellness last forever. Don't just focus on making the customer FEEL GOOD, focus on getting the client results.

Do they want to clear up their skin, tone their body, reduce stress? What is their END result? By helping the client set wellness goals, you become a necessity and NOT an option.

⇓

LAW #6: Working Without a Plan

When you fail to plan, you are planning to fail. You must have all types of plans from marketing plans to profit plans, and know how they all work together.

The marketing plan will get the client in the door, but if you don't have a profit plan, how do you know whether or not what you are doing is profitable? There are many spas that have gone out of business for not knowing their numbers; and not having a plan.

⇓

LAW #7: Not Focused on Retention and Referrals

Customers are the lifeblood of any business. The mass majority of customers have a minimum of 2 – 5 friends or relatives that have similar spending habits as they do.

When you focus obsessively on being FAR better than average and even go so far as to ASK your clients for referrals, and provide them with special perks and treatments, you not only get to retain your current client, but they will soon be sending you more than you can handle.

It is proof that people ONLY tell stories when an experience is horrible or when an experience is OVER-the-top great. You KNOW which category YOU want to be in.

⇩

LAW #8: Jack of All Trades

Wearing TOO many hats in your salon not only cannibalizes your time, but it also signals your team that you don't need them.

When you delegate, you empower and you equip. When you try to do it all, you weaken. When you are tired, there is no one that can or is willing to step into your exhausted shoes.

Set the standard up front that YOUR spa is a TEAM effort and your employees will follow suit.

LAW #9: Continuously Investing Your Staff, Your Salon and Yourself...

It is Biblical that you REAP what you sow. You should continuously be investing in the growth, education, and stability of your staff, your salon and yourself.

The best is NEVER good enough. As long as you put back into your business a portion of what you make consistently.

Invest towards recognition programs for both your clients and employees, as well as education for you and your employees.

With these investments, your spa won't miss a beat come rain or shine.

And let the Spa say...AMEN!

Thanks for Reading!

For more information about my mentorship program, books, and events, visit my website at:

https://candaceholyfield.com

Acknowledgments

Kay Williams
@theskintherapystudio

London Spears
@ls_massage_therapy_llc

Tyra Henderson
@clevelandsgiftedhands

Sparkle Davis CMT 360
Therapeutic Massage

Nykol Wynn @tenderly4you

Patrice Smith @shoploveshae

Jaleel Gilmore @imassage4la

Candice Cummings CMT
@2thepointmt

@iamkorirusse @maconperfections

Krrilyn Brown @wellendeavors

Kwame Huntley
@bellabodyworksmtw

Nicole J Loc educator
@adibynicolej Youtube: Salon Noa TV

@yourskinblis @misstennessee1

Shirley Mabern - Memphis, TN

@salon_zen

@justlikepaint

Anothy Parker - Memphis, TN

83 ... Acknowledgments

@millionairemassagedutches

Raven Little RN CPR classes
Vsteam Lounge @ravenlittlernpllc

Acknowledgments ... 84

The End

Made in United States
North Haven, CT
07 November 2021

10910258R00056